Dr. Sebi juicing recipes book

DR. SEBI JUICING RECIPE BOOK

Natural Alkaline Juices to Heal, reduce Inflammation, detoxify and Revitalize Your Body.

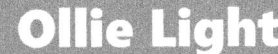

Dr. Sebi juicing recipes book

Copyrights/Disclaimer

© [2024] by [Ollie light]. All rights reserved.

This book cannot be duplicated, saved in a retrieval system, or transmitted in any way, whether it be electronically, mechanically, by photocopying, recording, or by any other means, without the publisher's prior written consent.

This book, "Dr. Sebi Juicing Recipe Book," contains information that is intended solely for educational and informative reasons. This book's recipes, recommendations, and advice are not meant to replace a doctor's advice, diagnosis, or course of treatment. When in doubt about a medical problem, never hesitate to consult your doctor or another trained healthcare professional. Never ignore medical advice from professionals or put off getting treatment because of what this book says.

About the Author

Ollie Light is a chef and mother who is passionate about healthy eating and living. After going through a difficult divorce, she found solace in the kitchen and has since developed a full-fledged culinary career. Ollie runs a catering business that sources local ingredients and incorporates flavors from around the world. She also teaches community cooking classes and donates her skills to charity events and food banks. Ollie has a dream of writing inspiring books and publishing her own cookbook to make nutritious food more accessible. She is living proof that pursuing your passion can lead to fulfillment and uses her gifts to nurture and inspire others.

Dr. Sebi juicing recipes book

Contents of the Book

INTRODUCTION
    The Dr. Sebi Alkaline Diet Approach
    Benefits of Juicing for Detox and Health
    How to Use This Book?
Chapter 1
    Juicing for Detoxification
    Green Power Detox Juice
    Cleansing Cucumber & Celery Juice
    Alkaline Lemon-Ginger Cleanse
    Detoxifying Kale & Dandelion Juice
Chapter 2
    Anti-Inflammatory Juices
    Understanding Inflammation and Its Impact
    Turmeric & Pineapple Inflammation Fighter
    Beetroot & Carrot Anti-Inflammatory Juice
    Ginger Citrus Immunity Booster
    Aloe Vera & Apple Healer Juice
CHAPTER 3
    Energy-Boosting Juices
    Understanding Energy and Nutrition
    Energizing Green Apple & Spinach Juice
    Vitality-Boosting Citrus & Parsley Juice
    Rejuvenating Watermelon & Mint Juice
    Sweet Potato & Ginger Morning Juice

Dr. Sebi juicing recipes book

Chapter 4
   Immune System Support Juices
   The Role of Nutrition in Immune Health
   Citrus & Berries Immune Power
   Elderberry & Grapefruit Immune Elixir
   Immune Strengthening Mango-Turmeric Juice
   Antioxidant-Rich Blueberry & Plum Juice

Chapter 5
   Weight Management & Metabolism Juices
   How Juicing Supports Weight Management and Metabolism
   The Natural Approach to Weight Management
   Metabolism-Boosting Cucumber & Lemon Juice
   Fat-Burning Apple, Kale & Cayenne Juice
   Slimming Papaya & Fennel Juice
   Weight-Loss Watercress & Lime Juice

Chapter 6
   Skin & Hair Health Juices
   How Juicing Supports Skin & Hair Health
   Glowing Skin Carrot & Orange Juice
   Radiant Skin Cucumber & Aloe Juice
   Hydrating Coconut Water & Cucumber Juice
   Hair-Nourishing Avocado & Cucumber Juice

Chapter 7
   Juices for Heart Health
   How Juicing Supports Heart Health
   Heart-Healthy Beet & Spinach Juice

Dr. Sebi juicing recipes book

- Cholesterol-Lowering Ginger & Apple Juice
- Blood Pressure Balancing Carrot & Celery Juice
- Cardiovascular Strength Blueberry & Pomegranate Juice

Chapter 8
- Juicing for Longevity
- The Science Behind Juicing for Longevity
- Longevity-Boosting Alkaline Green Juice
- Anti-Aging Watermelon & Cucumber Juice
- Brain Health Walnut & Blackberry Juice
- Youthful Glow Alkaline Juice Blend

Chapter 9
- Herbs & Alkaline Ingredients for Juicing
- Tips & Best Practices for Juicing
- How to Store and Serve Juices
- Living a Dr. Sebi Lifestyle for Long-Term Health
- Final Thoughts on Juicing and Holistic Health

INTRODUCTION

In this ever-evolving world where processed foods and synthetic chemicals dominate our diets, the Dr. Sebi Alkaline Diet approach offers a beacon of hope for those seeking true health and healing. This lifestyle is not merely a diet; it's a comprehensive, holistic approach to revitalize the body, mind, and spirit by harmonizing with nature's most nourishing gifts. Rooted in the ancient wisdom of plant-based living and the science of cellular health, this way of eating supports the body's natural ability to heal itself. The foods we consume directly impact our cellular function, immune system, and overall well-being. Thus, the foods promoted in the Dr. Sebi Alkaline Diet are carefully chosen to foster an environment where disease cannot thrive, allowing the body to reach its optimum level of health.

The purpose of this book is to not only introduce you to this powerful way of life but also to provide practical, simple, and nourishing recipes that align with the principles of the alkaline diet. Each meal, drink, and snack featured here is designed to nourish your cells, alkalize your system, and bring about vibrant health. Whether you're just starting your journey or have been following an alkaline diet for some time, this book serves as a resource to inspire and guide you. Remember, the goal isn't just to follow a restrictive diet but to transition into a lifestyle where health and balance are paramount. You will find a variety of recipes that are delicious and easy to prepare, making the alkaline lifestyle accessible and enjoyable for everyone.

The Dr. Sebi Alkaline Diet Approach

Dr. Sebi alkaline is built on the fundamental idea that the body operates best in an alkaline state. When our internal environment becomes too acidic, it creates a breeding ground for disease, inflammation, and dysfunction. By consuming alkaline foods, we can help the body maintain a pH balance that promotes optimal health. This is the essence of Dr. Sebi's teaching: disease cannot thrive in an alkaline environment, but it flourishes in acidity. The human body is made up of trillions of cells, and when these cells are nourished with the right nutrients, they can function at their highest capacity. Dr. Sebi believed that most modern diseases, such as diabetes, high blood pressure, and even cancer, stem from a disruption in this delicate balance.

The alkaline diet prioritizes natural, non-hybrid, plant-based foods that are free from artificial additives and chemicals. The focus is on fruits, vegetables, grains, and herbs that are closest to their natural state, unaltered by human intervention. Hybrid and genetically modified foods are avoided because they disrupt the body's natural healing processes. Instead, the diet emphasizes whole, organic foods that are rich in vital nutrients. By eating in alignment with nature, we allow the body to return to its original state of health. This means reducing or eliminating foods that are high in acidity, such as processed sugars, animal products, and refined grains, and replacing them with alkaline-forming foods.

Benefits of Juicing for Detox and Health

Juicing plays a vital role in the Dr. Sebi Alkaline Diet, offering a powerful way to flood the body with nutrients while aiding in detoxification. Freshly made juices from alkaline-approved fruits and vegetables provide a concentrated source of vitamins, minerals, and antioxidants that can be absorbed quickly by the body. Juicing allows us to consume a higher volume of nutrients than we typically could through eating alone. This is especially beneficial when detoxifying the body, as the nutrients from these juices help cleanse the blood, tissues, and organs, enabling the body to eliminate toxins more efficiently.

One of the key benefits of juicing is its ability to hydrate the body on a deep cellular level. Many people suffer from chronic dehydration without even realizing it, and juicing helps to replenish the body's water supply while providing it with essential nutrients. Juicing also allows the digestive system to rest. Since the fiber is removed in the juicing process, the body can focus on absorbing nutrients instead of breaking down food. This makes juicing an ideal practice during times of detoxification, as it supports the body's natural cleansing processes. It's also a fantastic way to give your immune system a boost, reduce inflammation, and increase energy levels.

How to Use This Book?

This book is designed as your companion on the journey to achieving vibrant health through the principles of the Dr. Sebi Alkaline Diet. Whether you are a beginner or have been following this lifestyle for a while, the recipes and guidance provided here will serve as a practical resource to support your transition into a fully alkaline way of living. Each recipe is carefully curated to include ingredients that align with Dr. Sebi's dietary guidelines, ensuring that every meal you prepare will help nourish your body and promote healing.

Dr. Sebi juicing recipes book

We begin by explaining the fundamentals of the alkaline diet, its benefits, and how to make a smooth transition from an acidic, processed diet to one that is natural, alkaline, and healing. The book then progresses through various sections, offering a variety of meal ideas from breakfast to dinner, along with snacks and beverages that can easily fit into your daily routine. You will also find a section dedicated to juicing, which plays a critical role in detoxifying the body and providing concentrated nutrients.

Additionally, this book includes tips for stocking your kitchen with alkaline ingredients, suggestions for essential kitchen tools, and strategies for maintaining consistency as you incorporate these new habits into your life. The transition to an alkaline diet is a transformative process, and this book is here to make that journey as seamless and enjoyable as possible. Use it as a guide, an inspiration, and a stepping stone toward better health. You'll find that once you embrace the alkaline lifestyle, your energy levels increase, your skin glows, and you experience a deeper sense of well-being. By the end, you'll have all the tools you need to nourish your body, heal from within, and live vibrantly.

Dr. Sebi juicing recipes book

Chapter 1

Juicing for Detoxification

Juicing is one of the most potent and effective ways to detoxify the body, particularly when aligned with the principles of Dr. Sebi's Alkaline Diet. Detoxification is essential for cellular health and overall vitality, and juicing offers a concentrated source of natural nutrients that the body can easily absorb and utilize. The purpose of detoxing through juicing is to cleanse the body at a cellular level, removing accumulated toxins, heavy metals, and acidic waste that compromise health. In doing so, you provide your cells with the optimal environment to regenerate, rejuvenate, and maintain balance.

At the heart of Dr. Sebi's teachings is the idea that the body is designed to heal itself, but it requires the right conditions. These conditions can only be achieved when the body is free from toxins and nourished with alkaline-forming, plant-based nutrients. Juicing is a powerful tool in this process, as it floods the body with essential vitamins, minerals, and antioxidants while giving the digestive system a rest. This rest allows the body to focus its energy on detoxifying and repairing itself rather than processing heavy, dense, or toxic foods.

Green Power Detox Juice

Servings: 2 | Preparation Time: 10 minutes | Total Time: 10 minutes

Ingredients:

2 cups kale, chopped

1 green apple, cored and sliced

1 cucumber, peeled and chopped

1/2 lemon, peeled

1-inch piece of fresh ginger

1 cup water

Directions:

1. Prepare the Ingredients: Chop the kale, cucumber, and green apple into manageable pieces for your juicer or blender. Make sure to peel the lemon and ginger to enhance the smoothness of your juice.

2. Blend or Juice: Combine all ingredients in a blender or juicer, adding 1 cup of water. Blend until smooth, and strain through a fine mesh sieve or cheesecloth if you prefer a clearer juice.

3. Serve: Pour the juice into glasses and enjoy immediately to maximize freshness and nutrient intake.

Nutritional Benefit:

Kale is rich in vitamins A, C, and K, which bolster the immune system. Cucumber hydrates while ginger aids digestion, making this juice an excellent detox choice.

Nutritional Values (per serving):

Calories: 90 | Carbohydrates: 20g | Protein: 3g | Fat: 0g | Fiber: 4g | Sugar: 11g

Cooking Tips:

For an even smoother juice, consider straining it multiple times to remove excess pulp.

Chill the ingredients beforehand for a refreshing cold drink.

Cleansing Cucumber & Celery Juice

Servings: 2 | Preparation Time: 10 minutes | Total Time: 10 minutes

Ingredients:

2 cucumbers, peeled and chopped

3 stalks of celery, chopped

1/2 lemon, peeled

1 green apple, cored and sliced

1/2 cup water

Directions:

1. Prepare the Ingredients: Chop the cucumbers and celery into small pieces. Core and slice the apple, and peel the lemon to make the juice smoother and more palatable.

2. Juice or Blend: Add all ingredients into your juicer or blender with the water. Blend until smooth, and strain if you prefer a pulp-free juice.

3. Serve: Pour into glasses and enjoy right away for optimal flavor and freshness

Nutritional Benefit: Cucumbers and celery are low in calories and high in water content, promoting hydration. The lemon adds vitamin C, enhancing detoxification.

Nutritional Values (per serving): Calories: 60 | Carbohydrates: 12g | Protein: 2g | Fat: 0g | Fiber: 2g | Sugar: 7g

Cooking Tips:

If using a blender, blending the ingredients longer can help break down the fibers for a smoother texture.

For added flavor, you can throw in a handful of fresh mint or a pinch of salt.

Dr. Sebi juicing recipes book

Alkaline Lemon-Ginger Cleanse

Servings: 2 | Preparation Time: 5 minutes | Total Time: 5 minutes

Ingredients:

2 cups warm water

Juice of 1 lemon

1-inch piece of fresh ginger, grated

1-2 tsp raw honey (optional)

Directions:

1. Combine Ingredients: In a large glass, mix warm water with freshly squeezed lemon juice and grated ginger. If desired, add raw honey for sweetness.

2. Stir Well: Use a spoon to mix thoroughly, ensuring the ginger is evenly distributed.

3. Serve: Drink this cleansing mixture warm in the morning to kick start your metabolism.

Nutritional Benefit:

Lemon aids digestion and detoxification, while ginger has anti-inflammatory properties that can soothe the stomach.

Nutritional Values (per serving): Calories: 50 | Carbohydrates: 11g | Protein: 1g | Fat: 0g | Fiber: 1g | Sugar: 6g

Cooking Tips:

For an extra boost, consider adding a dash of cayenne pepper or a few mint leaves.

Make a larger batch and refrigerate for up to 2 days, just remember to shake before consuming.

Detoxifying Kale & Dandelion Juice

Servings: 2 | Preparation Time: 10 minutes | Total Time: 10 minutes

Ingredients:

1 cup kale, chopped

1 cup dandelion greens, washed and chopped

1 green apple, cored and sliced

1/2 lemon, peeled

1-inch cucumber, chopped

1 cup water

Directions:

1. Prepare the Greens: Wash the kale and dandelion greens thoroughly to remove any grit. Chop the apple and cucumber for easier blending.

2. Juice or Blend: Combine all ingredients in a blender or juicer, adding the water. Blend until smooth, and strain if you desire a juice without pulp.

3. Serve: Pour into glasses and consume immediately to enjoy the maximum health benefits.

Nutritional Benefit:

Dandelion greens are packed with nutrients and have detoxifying properties, while kale provides essential vitamins. This juice is a great way to support liver health.

Nutritional Values (per serving): Calories: 85 | Carbohydrates: 18g | Protein: 4g | Fat: 0g | Fiber: 3g | Sugar: 5g

Cooking Tips:

Dandelion greens can be bitter, so balance with a sweeter apple if preferred.

Dr. Sebi juicing recipes book

Chapter 2

Anti-Inflammatory Juices

Understanding Inflammation and Its Impact

In the pursuit of optimal health and wellness, inflammation often takes center stage as a crucial factor impacting our overall well-being. Chronic inflammation is linked to numerous health issues, including heart disease, arthritis, and autoimmune disorders. The good news is that certain juices can help combat this inflammation and restore balance to the body. Anti-inflammatory juices harness the power of natural, nutrient-dense ingredients that are rich in antioxidants, vitamins, and minerals, working synergistically to reduce inflammation and promote healing.

Inflammation is a natural response of the body's immune system to injury, infection, or harmful stimuli. While acute inflammation can be beneficial, chronic inflammation can lead to a range of health problems. Diet plays a significant role in managing inflammation, and incorporating anti-inflammatory juices into your daily routine can be an effective way to support your body's natural defenses. Juicing allows for the concentrated intake of anti-inflammatory compounds that can be easily absorbed, providing immediate benefits to your cells.

Turmeric & Pineapple Inflammation Fighter

Servings: 2 | Preparation Time: 10 minutes | Total Time: 10 minutes

Ingredients:

1 cup fresh pineapple chunks

1/2 tsp fresh turmeric root, peeled

1/2 lemon, peeled

1-inch piece fresh ginger

1/4 tsp black pepper (enhances turmeric absorption)

1/2 cup coconut water

Directions:

1. Prep the Ingredients: Chop the pineapple into chunks, peel the turmeric and ginger, and slice the lemon.

2. Blend or Juice: Add all the ingredients into a blender or juicer, including the coconut water. Blend until smooth and strain for a cleaner texture if desired.

3. Serve: Enjoy immediately with a sprinkle of black pepper to maximize the bioavailability of the curcumin in turmeric.

Nutritional Benefit:

Turmeric is a powerful anti-inflammatory agent, and when paired with black pepper, its active compound curcumin becomes more bioavailable. Pineapple adds bromelain, which further reduces inflammation, especially in joints.

Nutritional Values (per serving): Calories: 100 | Carbohydrates: 23g | Protein: 1g | Fat: 0g | Fiber: 2g | Sugar: 20g

Cooking Tips:

Turmeric can be potent in flavor, so adjust the amount based on personal preference.

Using coconut water instead of regular water adds electrolytes, perfect for post-workout recovery.

Dr. Sebi juicing recipes book

Beetroot & Carrot Anti-Inflammatory Juice

Servings: | 2 Preparation Time: 10 minutes | Total Time: 10 minutes

Ingredients:

2 medium beets, peeled and chopped

3 large carrots, peeled

1 green apple, cored and sliced

1/2 lemon, peeled

1/2-inch piece of fresh ginger

Directions:

1. Prepare the Veggies: Peel and chop the beets and carrots into small pieces for easy blending. Core and slice the apple and peel the ginger.

2. Juice or Blend: Add all the ingredients into your juicer or blender. If using a blender, add a bit of water for smoother blending and strain after blending if you prefer less pulp.

3. Serve: Pour the juice into glasses and enjoy immediately for maximum nutrient retention.

Nutritional Benefit:

Beetroot contains betaines, known for their anti-inflammatory and detoxifying properties, while carrots provide beta-carotene, which helps fight oxidative stress.

Nutritional Values (per serving): Calories: 90 | Carbohydrates: 22g | Protein: 2g | Fat: 0g | Fiber: 3g | Sugar: 15g

Cooking Tips:

Beets can be overpowering, so adjust the apple or carrot ratio to balance the sweetness.

Ginger Citrus Immunity Booster

Servings: 2 | Preparation Time: 5 minutes | Total Time: 5 minutes

Ingredients:

2 oranges, peeled

1 lemon, peeled

1-inch piece of fresh ginger

1 tsp raw honey (optional)

Directions:

1. Prep the Citrus: Peel the oranges and lemon, and slice the ginger into smaller pieces for easier blending or juicing.

2. Juice or Blend: Add all the ingredients to your juicer or blender. If blending, strain the mixture afterward for a smoother finish.

3. Serve: Pour the juice into glasses and stir in raw honey if you'd like a touch of sweetness. Enjoy immediately.

Nutritional Benefit:

Ginger is renowned for its anti-inflammatory properties, particularly in the digestive system, while the citrus fruits provide a hefty dose of vitamin C for immune support.

Nutritional Values (per serving):

Calories: 80 | Carbohydrates: 21g | Protein: 1g | Fat: 0g | Fiber: 2g | Sugar: 16g

Cooking Tips:

For an added kick, consider adding a pinch of cayenne pepper to the mix.

You can make this juice the night before for a quick immune boost in the morning.

Dr. Sebi juicing recipes book

Aloe Vera & Apple Healer Juice

Servings: 2 | Preparation Time: 5 minutes | Total Time: 5 minutes

Ingredients:

1 cup aloe vera juice (store-bought or fresh)

2 green apples, cored and sliced

1/2 lemon, peeled

Directions:

1. Prep the Ingredients: Core and slice the apples and peel the lemon.

2. Juice or Blend: Add the apples and lemon to your juicer or blender. Mix with aloe vera juice after juicing or blending. Strain if needed.

3. Serve: Pour into glasses and enjoy the refreshing, healing properties of aloe and apple.

Nutritional Benefit:

Aloe vera is known for its anti-inflammatory and digestive benefits. Apple adds fiber and vitamin C, contributing to gut health and immune function.

Nutritional Value (per serving): Calories: 70 | Carbohydrates: 18g | Protein: 1g | Fat: 0g | Fiber: 4g | Sugar: 12g

Cooking Tips:

Aloe can have a slightly bitter taste, so adjusting the apple ratio can help balance it.

Use fresh aloe gel if available for a more potent, unprocessed juice.

Dr. Sebi juicing recipes book

CHAPTER 3

Energy-Boosting Juices

In our fast-paced world, maintaining high energy levels is essential for optimal performance in daily life. Many individuals struggle with fatigue and low energy, often turning to caffeine or sugary snacks for a quick pick-me-up. However, a more sustainable and healthier approach to boosting energy is through the consumption of nutrient-dense, energy-boosting juices. These vibrant beverages harness the power of fruits and vegetables, providing the body with essential vitamins, minerals, and antioxidants that not only invigorate the spirit but also support long-lasting vitality.

Understanding Energy and Nutrition

Energy in the body is derived from the foods we consume, which provide the fuel necessary for cellular processes, physical activity, and mental clarity. Nutrient-rich foods, particularly those high in complex carbohydrates, healthy fats, and proteins, play a crucial role in maintaining energy levels. Juices made from fresh, whole foods can enhance nutrient absorption, making it easier for the body to access the energy it needs without the crash associated with processed snacks.

Energizing Green Apple & Spinach Juice

Servings: 2 | Preparation Time: 10 minutes | Total Time: 10 minutes

Ingredients:

2 green apples, cored and chopped

1 cup fresh spinach

1/2 cucumber, chopped

1/2 lemon, peeled

1-inch piece of fresh ginger

Directions:

1. Prep the Ingredients: Core and chop the apples, and slice the cucumber and ginger. Peel the lemon for juicing.

2. Juice or Blend: Add all ingredients to your juicer or blender. If blending, include a splash of water for easier blending and strain afterward if desired.

3. Serve: Pour the juice into glasses and enjoy immediately for the best flavor and nutrient retention.

Nutritional Benefit:

Green apples provide antioxidants and vitamins, while spinach is rich in iron and magnesium, promoting energy and vitality.

Nutritional Values (per serving): Calories: 80 | Carbohydrates: 20g | Protein: 2g | Fat: 0g | Fiber: 4g | Sugar: 10g

Cooking Tips:

For a sweeter juice, you can add an extra apple or a splash of honey.

Experiment by adding other greens like kale for additional nutrients.

Vitality-Boosting Citrus & Parsley Juice

Servings: 2 | Preparation Time: 10 minutes | Total Time: 10 minutes

Ingredients:

2 oranges, peeled

1 grapefruit, peeled

1/2 lemon, peeled

1/4 cup fresh parsley

1-inch piece of ginger

Directions:

1. Prep the Ingredients: Peel the oranges, grapefruit, and lemon, and slice the ginger for juicing.

2. Juice or Blend: Combine all ingredients in your juicer or blender. If blending, add a little water for a smoother consistency and strain if desired.

3. Serve: Pour the juice into glasses and enjoy fresh for the best health benefits.

Nutritional Benefit:

Citrus fruits are excellent sources of vitamin C, enhancing immune function, while parsley adds vitamins K and A for added health benefits.

Nutritional Values (per serving): Calories: 90 | Carbohydrates: 22g | Protein: 2g | Fat: 0g | Fiber: 3g | Sugar: 18g

Cooking Tips:

Adjust the citrus ratio to suit your taste; more lemon can enhance the tartness.

Add a splash of coconut water for added hydration and a tropical twist.

Rejuvenating Watermelon & Mint Juice

Servings: 2 Preparation Time: 5 minutes Total Time: 5 minutes

Ingredients:

4 cups watermelon, cubed and seeded

1/4 cup fresh mint leaves

1 lime, peeled

Directions:

1. Prep the Ingredients: Cube the watermelon and peel the lime for juicing.

2. Juice or Blend: Add the watermelon, mint leaves, and lime to your juicer or blender. Blend until smooth; strain if you prefer a smoother texture.

3. Serve: Pour into glasses and garnish with a sprig of mint for a refreshing touch.

Nutritional Benefit:

Watermelon is hydrating and rich in vitamins A and C, while mint aids digestion and adds a refreshing flavor.

Nutritional Values (per serving): Calories: 70 | Carbohydrates: 18g | Protein: 1g | Fat: 0g | Fiber: 1g | Sugar: 15g

Cooking Tips:

Freeze some watermelon cubes ahead of time for a chilled version that requires no ice.

For a more invigorating taste, add a slice of fresh ginger.

Sweet Potato & Ginger Morning Juice

Servings: 2 | Preparation Time: 10 minutes Total Time: 10 minutes

Ingredients:

1 medium sweet potato, peeled and chopped

1-inch piece of fresh ginger, peeled

1 orange, peeled

1/2 lemon, peeled

1/2 cup water

Directions:

1. Prep the Ingredients: Chop the sweet potato and peel the ginger, orange, and lemon for juicing.

2. Juice or Blend: Combine all ingredients in your juicer or blender, adding water to aid blending. If using a blender, strain afterward for a smoother texture.

3. Serve: Pour into glasses and enjoy this warming juice for breakfast or a midmorning snack.

Nutritional Benefit:

Sweet potatoes are rich in beta-carotene and fiber, supporting healthy digestion and eye health, while ginger adds anti-inflammatory properties.

Nutritional Values (per serving): Calories: 100 | Carbohydrates: 24g | Protein: 2g | Fat: 0g | Fiber: 4g | Sugar: 6g

Cooking Tips:

For a creamier texture, consider adding a splash of coconut milk.

You can also use cooked sweet potatoes for a sweeter taste and easier blending.

Dr. Sebi juicing recipes book

Chapter 4

Immune System Support Juices

Our immune system is the body's first line of defense against infections, viruses, and harmful bacteria. In today's world, with environmental pollutants, stress, and various lifestyle factors weakening our natural immunity, it is more important than ever to support and strengthen the immune system through proper nutrition. One of the most effective and delicious ways to achieve this is by incorporating immune boosting juices into your daily routine. These vibrant, nutrient-packed juices are filled with vitamins, minerals, antioxidants, and phytonutrients that fortify the body's natural defenses, allowing you to maintain optimal health and vitality.

The Role of Nutrition in Immune Health

Your immune system relies on a constant supply of essential nutrients to function efficiently. Certain vitamins and minerals, particularly vitamins C, A, D, E, and zinc, play critical roles in the maintenance and operation of the immune system. Antioxidants, which are naturally found in fruits and vegetables, also help neutralize harmful free radicals, reducing oxidative stress and inflammation—two factors that can compromise immune function. By juicing nutrient-dense fruits and vegetables, you ensure that your body receives these powerful immune-supporting compounds in a highly absorbable and concentrated form.

Citrus & Berries Immune Power

Servings: 2 | Preparation Time: 10 minutes | Total Time: 10 minutes

Ingredients:

2 oranges, peeled

1/2 cup mixed berries (blueberries, strawberries, raspberries)

1/2 lemon, peeled

1 tablespoon honey (optional)

Directions:

1. Prep the Ingredients: Peel the oranges and lemon, and gather your mixed berries.

2. Juice or Blend: Add the citrus and berries to your juicer or blender. If using a blender, add a splash of water or juice for easier blending. Strain if desired.

3. Serve: Pour into glasses and enjoy the fresh, tangy flavor, optionally drizzling a bit of honey on top for sweetness.

Nutritional Benefit:

Citrus fruits are loaded with vitamin C, which boosts immunity and skin health, while berries are rich in antioxidants that help fight free radicals in the body.

Nutritional Values (per serving): Calories: 110 | Carbohydrates: 26g | Protein: 2g | Fat: 0g | Fiber: 4g | Sugar: 18g

Cooking Tips:

For a stronger berry flavor, adjust the ratio of berries to citrus.

Add a few ice cubes before blending for a chilled, refreshing version.

Dr. Sebi juicing recipes book

Elderberry & Grapefruit Immune Elixir

Servings: 2 | Preparation Time: 10 minutes | Total Time: 10 minutes

Ingredients:

1/2 cup elderberry syrup (store-bought or homemade)

2 grapefruits, peeled

1 tablespoon lemon juice

1 teaspoon grated fresh ginger

Directions:

1. Prep the Ingredients: Peel the grapefruits and gather the elderberry syrup and ginger.

2. Juice or Blend: Add the grapefruits, elderberry syrup, lemon juice, and grated ginger to your juicer or blender. Blend until smooth, straining if necessary.

3. Serve: Pour into glasses and drink immediately for the best immune supporting benefits.

Nutritional Benefit:

Elderberries are known for their antiviral properties, while grapefruit provides a high dose of vitamin C to strengthen the immune system.

Nutritional Values (per serving): Calories: 90 | Carbohydrates: 24g | Protein: 1g | Fat: 0g | Fiber: 3g | Sugar: 18g

Cooking Tips:

For a sweeter elixir, add a teaspoon of honey.

You can freeze the juice into ice cubes to make a refreshing immune-boosting ice tea.

Immune Strengthening Mango-Turmeric Juice

Servings: 2 | Preparation Time: 10 minutes | Total Time: 10 minutes

Ingredients:

1 ripe mango, peeled and chopped

1/2 orange, peeled

1/2 cup coconut water

1/2 teaspoon ground turmeric (or 1 inch piece fresh turmeric)

A pinch of black pepper (to activate turmeric)

Directions:

1. Prep the Ingredients: Peel and chop the mango and orange, and gather the coconut water and turmeric.

2. Juice or Blend: Add all ingredients into your blender or juicer, blending until smooth. If using fresh turmeric, grate it before adding. Strain if needed.

3. Serve: Pour the juice into glasses and drink fresh for the most benefits.

Nutritional Benefit:

Mango is rich in vitamins A and C, supporting immune health, while turmeric offers powerful anti-inflammatory properties, activated by the black pepper.

Nutritional Values (per serving): Calories: 120 | Carbohydrates: 28g | Protein: 2g | Fat: 1g | Fiber: 4g | Sugar: 24g

Cooking Tips:

Add a teaspoon of fresh lemon juice for an extra citrusy zing.

You can substitute coconut water with plain water if you prefer a less sweet flavor.

Antioxidant-Rich Blueberry & Plum Juice

Servings: 2 | Preparation Time: 10 minutes Total Time: 10 minutes

Ingredients:

1 cup fresh blueberries

2 ripe plums, pitted

1/2 cup water or coconut water

1 tablespoon fresh lime juice.

Directions:

1. Prep the Ingredients: Wash the blueberries and pit the plums. Gather your water or coconut water.

2. Juice or Blend: Add the blueberries, plums, and water into a blender or juicer. Blend until smooth and strain if necessary.

3. Serve: Pour into glasses and enjoy immediately, garnishing with a lime wedge if desired.

Nutritional Benefit:

Blueberries are packed with antioxidants that protect against oxidative stress, while plums aid digestion and provide a good source of vitamins A and C.

Nutritional Values (per serving): Calories: 100 | Carbohydrates: 24g | Protein: 1g | Fat: 0g | Fiber: 5g | Sugar: 18g

Cooking Tips:

You can freeze this juice in popsicle molds for a cool, antioxidant-rich treat.

Add a handful of spinach to the juice for an extra dose of greens without compromising the taste.

Dr. Sebi juicing recipes book

Chapter 5

Weight Management & Metabolism Juices

Weight management is a multifaceted journey that involves not only dietary choices but also lifestyle habits, physical activity, and metabolic health. One powerful, natural approach to managing weight is incorporating juices designed to rev up your metabolism, cleanse your body of toxins, and provide essential nutrients while keeping you full and energized. These juices are not about quick fixes or fad diets but focus on nourishing your body from the inside out, supporting sustainable weight loss and boosting overall metabolic health.

The beauty of juicing for weight management is that it allows you to flood your body with essential vitamins, minerals, and antioxidants, all while reducing calorie intake and promoting fat burning. When combined with a balanced alkaline diet, these juices can help regulate metabolism, control cravings, and improve digestive health key factors in achieving and maintaining a healthy weight.

How Juicing Supports Weight Management and Metabolism

Weight loss isn't just about cutting calories; it's about optimizing your body's ability to burn fat efficiently and maintain lean muscle mass. Juicing helps in the following ways:

1. Boosting Metabolism: Certain fruits and vegetables, particularly those rich in vitamin C, B vitamins, and minerals like magnesium, help improve metabolic function, allowing the

body to burn calories more effectively. Spices like cayenne pepper and ginger can also stimulate thermogenesis, the production of heat by the body induced by a single nutrient, a meal, a meal pattern or Drug.

2. Detoxifying the you desire a juice without pulp. Body: A sluggish metabolism is often tied to a buildup of toxins in the body, which can result in bloating, water retention, and weight gain. Juicing detoxifies the liver, kidneys, and digestive system, helping your body eliminate waste and reducing the toxic load, thus improving metabolic function.

3. Balancing Blood Sugar: When your blood sugar is stable, you're less likely to experience energy crashes or intense cravings for unhealthy foods. Juicing helps control blood sugar by providing slow-digesting fiber (when pulp is included) and nutrients that support insulin sensitivity, such as chromium and magnesium.

4. Suppressing Appetite: Drinking a nutrient-rich juice can help curb your appetite by providing essential nutrients that signal to your body that it's nourished, thus reducing the likelihood of overeating or snacking between meals.

The Natural Approach to Weight Management

Juicing for weight management and metabolism is not about restrictive dieting but nourishing your body with natural, whole ingredients that support fat-burning, detoxification, and metabolic health. By incorporating these vibrant, nutrient-dense juices into your daily routine, you can boost your metabolism, curb cravings, and support your weight loss journey in a sustainable, healthy way. With the right combination of ingredients, these juices offer a delicious and convenient way to fuel your body while achieving your health and fitness goals

Metabolism-Boosting Cucumber & Lemon Juice

Servings: 2 | Preparation Time: 10 minutes | Total Time: 10 minutes

Ingredients:

1 large cucumber, peeled

1 lemon, peeled

1/2-inch fresh ginger

1/2 cup water

1 teaspoon honey (optional)

Directions:

1. Prepare the Ingredients: Peel and chop the cucumber and lemon into smaller chunks for easier blending. Grate or slice the fresh ginger.

2. Blend or Juice: Add the cucumber, lemon, ginger, and water to your blender or juicer. Blend until smooth or juice if using a juicer. If blending, you can strain the mixture through a fine mesh sieve if you prefer a smoother texture.

3. Serve: Pour into a glass and stir in honey if you'd like a touch of sweetness. Drink immediately for the most refreshing and metabolism boosting effect.

Nutritional Benefit:

Cucumbers are hydrating and low in calories, while lemons are rich in vitamin C, aiding digestion and metabolism. Ginger further supports digestion and can help boost fat burning.

Nutritional Values (per serving): Calories: 35 | Carbohydrates: 8g | Protein: 1g | Fat: 0g | Fiber: 2g | Sugar: 4g

Cooking Tips:

Add a few ice cubes to the blender for an extra chilled effect.

For a detoxifying twist, include a few mint leaves.

Fat-Burning Apple, Kale & Cayenne Juice

Servings: 2 | Preparation Time: 10 minutes | Total Time: 10 minutes

Ingredients:

2 green apples, cored

1 cup kale leaves, stems removed

1/2 lemon, peeled

1/4 teaspoon cayenne pepper

1/2 cup water

Directions:

1. Prepare the Ingredients: Core the apples and remove the kale stems. Peel the lemon and gather the cayenne pepper.

2. Juice or Blend: Add the apples, kale, lemon, and water to your juicer or blender. Blend or juice until smooth. If blending, strain the mixture for a more juice-like consistency.

3. Add Cayenne: Once juiced, sprinkle in the cayenne pepper and stir thoroughly to ensure its well-mixed.

4. Serve: Pour into a glass, sip slowly, and feel the warmth of the cayenne kick in as it stimulates your metabolism.

Nutritional Benefit:

Apples are high in fiber and antioxidants, while kale is nutrient-dense and low in calories. Cayenne pepper is known to boost metabolism and help with fat-burning, making this juice an excellent option for those looking to support their weight loss goals.

Nutritional Values (per serving): Calories: 90 | Carbohydrates: 22g | Protein: 3g | Fat: 0g | Fiber: 5g | Sugar: 16g

Cooking Tips:

Adjust the cayenne to your heat tolerance—start with less and increase as desired.

Swap the water for coconut water for an added electrolyte boost.

Dr. Sebi juicing recipes book

Slimming Papaya & Fennel Juice

Servings:2 | Preparation Time:10 minutes | Total Time: 10 minutes

Dr. Sebi juicing recipes book

Ingredients:

1 cup papaya, peeled and cubed

1 small fennel bulb, trimmed

1/2-inch piece fresh ginger

1/2 cup coconut water

Directions:

1. Prepare the Ingredients: Peel and cube the papaya, trim the fennel bulb, and slice the ginger into small pieces.

2. Juice or Blend: Add the papaya, fennel, ginger, and coconut water to a blender or juicer. Blend until smooth or juice. Strain if you prefer a thinner consistency.

3. Serve: Pour the juice into a glass and enjoy its sweet, slightly herbal taste.

The lightness of the coconut water perfectly complements the natural sweetness of the papaya.

Nutritional Benefit:

Papaya contains digestive enzymes that help break down food, while fennel aids in digestion and helps reduce bloating, making this a great juice for anyone looking to feel lighter and more energized.

Nutritional Values (per serving): Calories: 80 | Carbohydrates: 19g | Protein: 1g | Fat: 0g | Fiber: 4g | Sugar: 13g

Cooking Tips:

For a spicier version, add a pinch of black pepper or cayenne.

Weight-Loss Watercress & Lime Juice

Servings:2 | Preparation Time:10 minutes | Total Time: 10 minutes

Ingredients:

1 cup fresh watercress leaves

1/2 lime, peeled

1/2 cucumber

1/2 cup cold water

Directions:

1. Prepare the Ingredients: Rinse the watercress, peel the lime, and chop the cucumber into smaller pieces.

2. Juice or Blend: Add the watercress, lime, cucumber, and cold water to your blender or juicer. Blend or juice until smooth, straining if desired for a more refined texture.

3. Serve: Pour the juice into a glass and enjoy its fresh, tangy flavor that leaves you feeling light and energized.

Nutritional Benefit:

Watercress is incredibly low in calories yet full of essential vitamins and minerals, while lime aids in digestion and helps flush toxins from the body. Cucumber adds hydration, making this a great juice for detoxing and weight loss.

Nutritional Values (per serving): Calories: 40 | Carbohydrates: 10g | Protein: 1g | Fat: 0g | Fiber: 3g | Sugar: 5g

Cooking Tips:

For an extra burst of flavor, add a handful of mint leaves.

Serve over ice for a super refreshing drink on a hot day.

Chapter 6

Skin & Hair Health Juices

Your skin and hair are reflections of your internal health, often showcasing how well-nourished and hydrated your body is. True beauty begins from within, and one of the most effective ways to nourish your skin and hair is through the power of juicing. Packed with vitamins, minerals, antioxidants, and hydration, skin and hair health juices can restore radiance, promote cell regeneration, strengthen hair follicles, and combat oxidative stress, leading to glowing skin and vibrant, healthy hair.

Juicing for skin and hair health taps into nature's purest sources of beauty: fruits, vegetables, and herbs that deliver potent nutrients directly to your cells. These juices flood the body with the antioxidants and anti-inflammatory compounds necessary for maintaining skin elasticity, combating premature aging, and preventing hair thinning or breakage.

How Juicing Supports Skin & Hair Health

1. Hydration: Both your skin and hair thrive on hydration. Juicing delivers high water content directly to your cells, keeping your skin plump and moisturized while promoting a healthy scalp for hair growth.

2. Antioxidants: Juices rich in antioxidants such as vitamins A, C, and E help fight free radical damage that can age the skin prematurely and weaken hair. These vitamins protect the skin from UV damage, pollution, and toxins while supporting healthy hair follicles.

3. Collagen Production: Vitamin C, in particular, is

crucial for collagen synthesis, the protein that provides structure to your skin and hair. Consuming vitamin C-rich juices helps keep your skin firm and your hair strong and lustrous.

4. **Anti-inflammatory Properties:** Inflammation can wreak havoc on both skin and hair, causing conditions like acne, eczema, psoriasis, and hair loss. Juices rich in anti-inflammatory compounds, such as those found in leafy greens, ginger, and turmeric, can soothe the skin and scalp, reducing irritation and redness.

5. **Nutrient Delivery:** Nutrients like biotin, silica, zinc, and omega-3 fatty acids are vital for hair growth and skin health. Juices provide an easy way to boost intake of these essential vitamins and minerals, helping to maintain a healthy complexion and prevent hair thinning.

Glowing Skin Carrot & Orange Juice

Servings: 2 | Preparation Time: 10 minutes | Total Time: 10 minutes

Ingredients:

4 medium carrots, peeled

2 large oranges, peeled

1/2-inch fresh ginger

1/2 cup water

Directions:

1. Prepare the Ingredients: Peel the carrots and oranges, and grate or slice the ginger.

2. Juice or Blend: Combine the carrots, oranges, ginger, and water in a juicer or blender. Blend until smooth or strain after blending if you prefer a thinner juice.

3. Serve: Pour into a glass and enjoy the radiant benefits of this skin-loving juice.

Nutritional Benefits:

Carrots are loaded with beta-carotene, which converts to vitamin A, promoting clear, healthy skin. Oranges are rich in vitamin C, supporting collagen production and brightening the skin.

Nutritional Values (per serving): Calories: 90 | Carbohydrates: 22g | Protein: 1g | Fat: 0g | Fiber: 4g | Sugar: 16g

Cooking Tips:

For an added detoxifying effect, squeeze in some fresh lemon juice.

Serve over ice for a cooling, refreshing drink.

Radiant Skin Cucumber & Aloe Juice

Servings: 2 | Preparation Time: 10 minutes | Total Time: 10 minutes

Ingredients:

1 large cucumber, peeled

1/4 cup aloe vera juice (fresh or store bought)

1/2 lime, peeled

1/2 cup cold water

Directions:

1. Prepare the Ingredients: Peel and chop the cucumber, and peel the lime.

2. Blend or Juice: Add the cucumber, aloe vera juice, lime, and water to a blender or juicer. Blend until smooth. Strain if desired for a smoother juice.

3. Serve: Pour into a glass and sip on this refreshing juice that hydrates and soothes your skin.

Nutritional Benefits:

Cucumbers are hydrating and high in silica, which supports skin elasticity, while aloe vera juice helps soothe and moisturize the skin, aiding in healing and hydration.

Nutritional Values (per serving): Calories: 50 | Carbohydrates: 12g | Protein: 0g | Fat: 0g | Fiber: 2g | Sugar: 6g

Cooking Tips:

Add a few mint leaves for a burst of freshness.

Chill the juice in the refrigerator for 10 minutes before serving for an extra refreshing drink.

Hydrating Coconut Water & Cucumber Juice

Servings:2 | Preparation Time 5 minutes | Total Time:5 minutes

Ingredients:

1 cup coconut water

1 large cucumber, peeled

1/4 lemon, peeled

Ice cubes (optional)

Directions:

1. Prepare the Ingredients: Peel and chop the cucumber and lemon.

2. Blend: Combine the coconut water, cucumber, and lemon in a blender. Blend until smooth.

3. Serve: Pour into a glass over ice cubes for an extra refreshing experience, and enjoy the hydrating benefits for your skin.

Nutritional Benefits:

Coconut water is rich in electrolytes, making it highly hydrating, while cucumber is full of water and skin-friendly antioxidants, helping to keep your skin plump and glowing.

Nutritional Values (per serving): Calories: 40 | Carbohydrates: 10g | Protein: 0g | Fat: 0g | Fiber: 1g | Sugar: 6g

Cooking Tips:

Add a slice of fresh lemon or a dash of sea salt for added flavor and minerals.

Use chilled coconut water to enhance the cooling effect.

Hair-Nourishing Avocado & Cucumber Juice

Servings: 2 | Preparation Time: 10 minutes | Total Time: 10 minutes

Ingredients:

1 ripe avocado

1 large cucumber, peeled

1/2 cup coconut milk

1/2 lime, peeled

Directions:

1. Prepare the Ingredients: Peel and pit the avocado, peel and chop the cucumber and lime.

2. Blend: Add the avocado, cucumber, coconut milk, and lime to a blender. Blend until smooth and creamy.

3. Serve: Pour the juice into a glass and enjoy the nourishing benefits for both your hair and skin.

Nutritional Benefit:

Avocados are rich in healthy fats, particularly monounsaturated fats, which help moisturize hair and skin. Cucumber provides hydration and silica, supporting hair strength and growth.

Nutritional Values (per serving): Calories: 150 | Carbohydrates: 10g | Protein: 2g | Fat: 12g | Fiber: 6g | Sugar: 4g

Cooking Tips:

For added sweetness, blend in a small apple or pear.

Serve chilled for a more refreshing experience.

Chapter 7

Juices for Heart Health

Heart health is one of the most critical aspects of overall wellness, and the choices we make daily can significantly influence the health of our cardiovascular system. Juicing provides an excellent way to ensure that your heart gets the nutrients it needs to function optimally. By incorporating heart-healthy fruits, vegetables, and herbs into your daily routine, you can reduce the risk of heart disease, lower blood pressure, manage cholesterol, and improve circulation.

Juices tailored for heart health are typically rich in antioxidants, potassium, magnesium, fiber, and heart-protective compounds like flavonoids and nitrates. These nutrients work in synergy to reduce inflammation, strengthen blood vessels, regulate blood pressure, and keep cholesterol levels in check. Let's explore how juicing can support your cardiovascular system and some of the most powerful ingredients that should be included in heart boosting juices.

How Juicing Supports Heart Health

1. Improves Circulation: Juicing ingredients such as beets and pomegranates are rich in nitrates, which convert to nitric oxide in the body. Nitric oxide helps to relax and dilate blood vessels, improving circulation and reducing blood pressure.

2. Reduces Inflammation: Inflammation is a key factor in the development of heart disease. Antioxidant-rich fruits and vegetables, like berries, leafy greens, and turmeric, help combat oxidative stress and reduce inflammation, protecting the heart and arteries.

3. Lowers Blood Pressure: Potassium Rich ingredients such as celery, spinach, and bananas help balance sodium levels in the body, thereby reducing high blood pressure, which is a major risk factor for heart disease.

4. Regulates Cholesterol Levels: Certain fruits, vegetables, and herbs, like apples, carrots, and garlic, contain soluble fiber and compounds that help to lower LDL cholesterol (bad cholesterol) and raise HDL cholesterol (good cholesterol).

5. Provides Essential Vitamins & Minerals: Vitamins C, E, K, magnesium, and folate are essential for heart health. These nutrients are abundant in fruits and vegetables like oranges, avocado, spinach, and kale, and they help maintain a healthy heart rhythm and support blood vessel integrity.

Heart-Healthy Beet & Spinach Juice

Servings: 2 | Preparation Time: 10 minutes | Total Time: 10 minutes

Ingredients:

2 medium beets, peeled

1 cup fresh spinach

1/2 cucumber, peeled

1/2 lemon, peeled

1/2 cup water

Directions:

1. Prepare the Ingredients: Peel and chop the beets, cucumber, and lemon. Rinse the spinach thoroughly.

2. Juice or Blend: Add the beets, spinach, cucumber, lemon, and water into a juicer or blender. Blend until smooth and strain if desired.

3. Serve: Pour the juice into a glass and enjoy the heart-healthy benefits of this vibrant juice.

Nutritional Benefit:

Beets are rich in nitrates, which help improve blood flow and lower blood pressure. Spinach adds fiber and iron, supporting overall cardiovascular health.

Nutritional Values (per serving): Calories: 80 | Carbohydrates: 18g | Protein: 3g | Fat: 0g | Fiber: 4g | Sugar: 10g

Cooking Tips:

Add a small piece of ginger for an extra anti-inflammatory boost.

Serve over ice for a refreshing touch.

Cholesterol-Lowering Ginger & Apple Juice

Servings: 2 | Preparation Time: 5 minutes | Total Time: 5 minutes

Ingredients:

2 medium apples, peeled and cored

1-inch fresh ginger

1/2 lemon, peeled

1/4 cup water

Directions:

1. Prepare the Ingredients: Peel and core the apples, peel the ginger and lemon.

2. Juice or Blend: Add the apples, ginger, lemon, and water into a juicer or blender. Blend until smooth and strain if needed.

3. Serve: Pour into a glass and enjoy this cholesterol-lowering juice packed with flavor.

Nutritional Benefit:

Ginger has anti-inflammatory properties that support heart health, while apples are high in soluble fiber, which helps reduce cholesterol levels.

Nutritional Values (per serving): Calories: 70 | Carbohydrates: 18g | Protein: 0g | Fat: 0g | Fiber: 3g | Sugar: 14g

Cooking Tips:

Use green apples for a tarter flavor and higher antioxidant content.

Add a dash of cinnamon for extra heart health benefits.

Blood Pressure Balancing Carrot & Celery Juice

Servings: 2 | Preparation Time: 10 minutes | Total Time: 10 minutes

Ingredients:

4 medium carrots, peeled

3 celery stalks

1/2 cucumber, peeled

1/2 lemon, peeled

Directions:

1. Prepare the Ingredients: Peel and chop the carrots and cucumber, and rinse the celery.

2. Juice or Blend: Add the carrots, celery, cucumber, and lemon into a juicer or blender. Blend until smooth. Strain for a thinner consistency, if desired.

3. Serve: Pour the juice into a glass and enjoy the blood pressure balancing benefits of this nutritious drink.

Nutritional Benefit:

Carrots are rich in beta-carotene, which supports overall heart health, while celery is high in potassium, which helps regulate blood pressure.

Nutritional Values (per serving): Calories: 50 | Carbohydrates: 12g | Protein: 1g | Fat: 0g | Fiber: 3g | Sugar: 8g

Cooking Tips:

Add a pinch of sea salt for added electrolytes.

Use organic celery for a stronger, more natural flavor.

Cardiovascular Strength Blueberry & Pomegranate Juice

Servings: 2 | Preparation Time: 5 minutes | Total Time: 5 minutes

Ingredients:

1/2 cup blueberries

1/2 cup pomegranate seeds

1/2 apple, peeled

1/4 cup water

Directions:

1. Prepare the Ingredients: Wash the blueberries and pomegranate seeds, and peel the apple.

2. Juice or Blend: Combine the blueberries, pomegranate seeds, apple, and water in a juicer or blender. Blend until smooth, and strain if desired.

3. Serve: Pour the juice into a glass and enjoy the cardiovascular strength benefits of this antioxidant-rich juice.

Nutritional Benefit:

Blueberries and pomegranates are rich in anthocyanin's, which help protect the heart from oxidative stress and improve blood circulation, supporting overall cardiovascular health.

Nutritional Values (per serving): Calories: 100 | Carbohydrates: 22g | Protein: 1g | Fat: 0g | Fiber: 5g | Sugar: 15g

Cooking Tips:

Use frozen blueberries for a thicker, smoothie-like texture.

Add a handful of spinach for extra nutrients without altering the flavor.

Chapter 8

Juicing for Longevity

Longevity isn't just about living a long life; It's about living a healthy long life with vitality, energy, and mental clarity. One of the most natural and effective ways to promote longevity is through juicing. This approach enables you to flood your body with concentrated doses of vitamins, minerals, and antioxidants, which work together to slow the aging process, boost cellular repair, and protect against chronic diseases. By integrating a wide range of nutrient-dense fruits, vegetables, and herbs into your daily juicing routine, you're giving your body the tools it needs to thrive well into old age.

The Science Behind Juicing for Longevity

The process of aging involves oxidative stress, cellular damage, inflammation, and gradual decline in bodily functions. However, many of these effects can be slowed down or even reversed with the right nutrition. Juicing allows the body to absorb large quantities of antioxidants and phytonutrients that neutralize harmful free radicals, repair damaged cells, and enhance the body's natural detoxification processes.

In particular, longevity-boosting juices focus on:

Reducing inflammation: Chronic inflammation accelerates aging and is linked to heart disease, diabetes, arthritis, and many other conditions. Anti-inflammatory ingredients like turmeric, ginger, and leafy greens help counteract this.

Enhancing cellular regeneration: Ingredients rich in vitamins A, C, and E, like berries, citrus, and carrots, promote cellular renewal and support healthy skin, organs, and immune function.

Detoxifying the body: A clean internal environment is crucial for longevity. Ingredients like cucumber, celery, and parsley help flush out toxins and support liver and kidney function.

Boosting the immune system: A strong immune system wards off infections and diseases. Juices packed with vitamin C, antioxidants, and adapt-genic herbs help keep the immune system robust.

Supporting brain health: Cognitive decline is a concern as we age. Nutrient-rich ingredients like blueberries, spinach, and avocado are excellent for boosting brain function and protecting against neurodegenerative diseases.

Longevity-Boosting Alkaline Green Juice

Servings: 2 | Preparation Time: 10 minutes | Total Time: 10 minutes

Ingredients:

1 cup spinach

1/2 cucumber, peeled

1 celery stalk

1/2 lemon, peeled

1/2 green apple, peeled

1 cup water

Directions:

1. Prepare the Ingredients: Wash the spinach and celery, and peel the cucumber, lemon, and apple.

2. Juice or Blend: Add the spinach, cucumber, celery, lemon, apple, and water to a juicer or blender. Blend until smooth and strain if you prefer a lighter consistency.

3. Serve: Pour into a glass and enjoy this longevity-boosting green juice as part of your daily health routine.

Nutritional Benefit:

This juice is rich in antioxidants from spinach and cucumber, while the alkalizing properties of lemon and celery help balance the body's pH, promoting better digestion and overall well-being.

Nutritional Values (per serving): Calories: 60 | Carbohydrates: 12g | Protein: 2g | Fat: 0g | Fiber: 3g | Sugar: 6g

Cooking Tips:

For an extra kick, add a small piece of ginger.

Anti-Aging Watermelon & Cucumber Juice

Servings: 2 | Preparation Time: 5 minutes | Total Time: 5 minutes

Ingredients:

2 cups watermelon, cubed

1/2 cucumber, peeled

1/2 lime, peeled

1/4 cup coconut water

Directions:

1. Prepare the Ingredients: Cube the watermelon, peel the cucumber, and prepare the lime.

2. Juice or Blend: Combine the watermelon, cucumber, lime, and coconut water in a blender or juicer. Blend until smooth and strain if desired.

3. Serve: Pour the juice into a glass and enjoy the refreshing, anti-aging benefits of this hydrating juice.

Nutritional Benefit:

Watermelon is packed with lycopene, which protects the skin from sun damage, while cucumber and coconut water help hydrate the skin, reducing the appearance of wrinkles.

Nutritional Values (per serving): Calories: 90 | Carbohydrates: 22g | Protein: 1g | Fat: 0g | Fiber: 2g | Sugar: 18g

Cooking Tips:

Add fresh mint leaves for a cooling flavor.

Serve over ice for a refreshing summer treat.

Brain Health Walnut & Blackberry Juice

Servings: 2 | Preparation Time: 10 minutes | Total Time: 10 minutes

Ingredients:

1/2 cup blackberries

1/4 cup walnuts

1/2 banana, frozen

1/2 cup almond milk

1/2 tsp cinnamon (optional)

Directions:

1. Prepare the Ingredients: Rinse the blackberries and gather the walnuts and frozen bananas.

2. Juice or Blend: Add the blackberries, walnuts, banana, almond milk, and cinnamon to a blender. Blend until smooth and creamy.

3. Serve: Pour the juice into a glass and enjoy this brain-boosting drink as a morning snack or post-workout recovery.

Nutritional Benefit:

Blackberries are high in antioxidants that protect the brain from aging, while walnuts provide omega-3 fatty acids, essential for brain health and cognitive function.

Nutritional Values (per serving): Calories: 120 | Carbohydrates: 16g | Protein: 3g | Fat: 5g | Fiber: 5g | Sugar: 10g

Cooking Tips:

For a thicker smoothie-like texture, add a handful of ice or use frozen blackberries.

Top with extra walnuts for a crunchy garnish.

Youthful Glow Alkaline Juice Blend

Servings: 2 | Preparation Time: 10 minutes | Total Time: 10 minutes

Ingredients:

1 cucumber, peeled

1 cup spinach

1/2 lemon, peeled

1/2 green apple

1/4 cup coconut water

Directions:

1. Prepare the Ingredients: Peel and chop the cucumber, lemon, and apple. Rinse the spinach thoroughly.

2. Juice or Blend: Add the cucumber, spinach, lemon, green apple, and coconut water to a juicer or blender. Blend until smooth and strain if desired.

3. Serve: Pour the juice into a glass and enjoy this skin-boosting, alkaline-rich drink.

Nutritional Benefit:

Cucumber and spinach are excellent for hydration, while lemon and green apple provide essential vitamins and antioxidants that help keep your skin looking youthful and vibrant.

Nutritional Values (per serving): Calories: 70 | Carbohydrates: 16g | Protein: 2g | Fat: 0g | Fiber: 4g | Sugar: 8g

Cooking Tips:

Add a teaspoon of chia seeds for a boost in fiber and omega-3s.

Serve chilled for maximum freshness and flavor.

Chapter 9

Herbs & Alkaline Ingredients for Juicing

In the world of alkaline juicing, herbs and specific alkaline ingredients offer a vast reservoir of nutrients, antioxidants, and medicinal properties. Juicing with herbs and alkaline vegetables not only enhances the nutritional value of your juices but also offers therapeutic benefits that support healing, detoxification, and overall wellness. Understanding the specific roles of these herbs and ingredients can empower you to make informed choices that bring your body back into balance, support your immune system, and promote longevity.

Juicing with herbs aligns with Dr. Sebi's holistic philosophy of using natural, non-hybrid, and alkaline foods to nourish the body and maintain its internal pH balance. Many herbs and alkaline foods are nature's most powerful healers, supporting detoxification, combating inflammation, and optimizing cellular health. Here's a closer look at key herbs and alkaline ingredients that can supercharge your juicing regimen.

1. **Burdock Root**: Burdock root is a powerful blood purifier and detoxifier. It helps to cleanse the liver and lymphatic system, making it an essential herb for those looking to support the body's natural detoxification processes. Rich in antioxidants, burdock root helps fight free radicals and reduce inflammation, both of which are crucial for maintaining alkaline balance. Its mildly sweet, earthy flavor blends well with root vegetable juices like carrots and beets.

Nutritional Information: Contains inulin (a type of fiber),

Dr. Sebi juicing recipes book

vitamin C, potassium, iron, and magnesium.

2. **Dandelion Greens:** Dandelion greens are a potent liver cleanser and diuretic, helping the body rid itself of toxins and excess water. This herb promotes healthy liver function and aids in detoxification, which is a key component of maintaining an alkaline environment in the body. Their slightly bitter taste can be balanced with sweet ingredients like apples or carrots.

Nutritional Information: High in vitamin A, vitamin C, calcium, iron, and potassium.

3. **Nettle Leaf:** Nettle leaf is revered for its anti-inflammatory and antihistamine properties. It is highly alkaline and packed with nutrients, making it an excellent herb for those seeking to support kidney health, combat inflammation, and strengthen the immune system. Nettle's mild, slightly grassy taste pairs well with green juices that include spinach, kale, and cucumber.

Nutritional Information: Rich in vitamins A, C, and K, as well as calcium, iron, and magnesium.

4. **Sarsaparilla:** Sarsaparilla is known for its powerful detoxifying and anti-inflammatory properties. It is particularly rich in iron, making it a fantastic herb for boosting energy levels and supporting the blood. In Dr. Sebi's teachings, sarsaparilla is often praised for its ability to cleanse the blood and promote a healthy immune system.

Nutritional Information: High in iron, antioxidants, and saponins (natural plant compounds that support immune health).

5. **Cilantro (Coriander):** Cilantro is a natural chelator, meaning it helps to remove heavy metals from the body, which can contribute to acidity. This powerful herb is also rich in antioxidants and promotes healthy digestion. The bright,

Dr. Sebi juicing recipes book

fresh flavor of cilantro can add a burst of vibrancy to green juices.

Nutritional Information: Contains vitamins A, C, K, and potassium.

6. Parsley: Parsley is a mild diuretic and a potent blood cleanser, helping to flush out toxins and support kidney health. Its high chlorophyll content makes it excellent for detoxifying the body and maintaining an alkaline ph.

Parsley's light, fresh flavor works well in green juices, adding a nutritional punch without overpowering other ingredients.

Nutritional Information: High in vitamins A, C, and K, and folate.

7. Alfalfa Grass: Alfalfa grass is a nutrient-dense herb packed with vitamins, minerals, and antioxidants. It helps to alkalize the body, cleanse the blood, and support digestive health. Alfalfa grass is also rich in enzymes that promote healthy digestion, making it a great addition to detoxifying juices.

Nutritional Information: Contains vitamins A, C, E, and K, as well as calcium, magnesium, and protein.

8. Elderberry: Elderberries are renowned for their immune boosting properties and are packed with antioxidants that fight free radicals and reduce oxidative stress. Elderberry juice is particularly beneficial during cold and flu season, offering natural antiviral and anti-inflammatory benefits.

Nutritional Information: High in vitamin C, antioxidants, and anthocyanin's.

9. Sea Moss (Irish Moss); Sea moss is a powerhouse of nutrients, providing the body with 92 of the 102 essential minerals it needs. This superfood is excellent for boosting energy, supporting thyroid health, and enhancing the immune system.

Its gel-like consistency makes it a perfect addition to smoothies or thick juices.

Nutritional Information: Contains iodine, calcium, magnesium, potassium, and vitamins A, C, E, and K.

10. Basil; Basil is more than just a culinary herb—it has potent medicinal properties. It supports digestion, reduces inflammation, and has antioxidant effects that help protect cells from damage. Basil is also known for its adaptogenic properties, helping the body manage stress, which is crucial for maintaining an alkaline state.

Nutritional Information: Rich in vitamins A, K, C, and iron.

11. Sage: Sage is another herb with powerful antioxidant properties. It helps reduce oxidative stress in the body, making it ideal for maintaining cellular health and slowing down the aging process. Sage also aids digestion and supports respiratory health.

Nutritional Information: High in vitamin K, antioxidants, and volatile oils that support immune health.

12. Mint: Mint is a soothing and refreshing herb that promotes healthy digestion and relieves nausea. It has natural cooling properties, making it great for calming the stomach and reducing inflammation. Mint's fresh, invigorating flavor pairs well with citrus fruits in juices.

Nutritional Information: Contains vitamin C, vitamin A, and magnesium.

13. Thyme: Thyme is a powerful antimicrobial herb that supports respiratory health, fights infections, and boosts the immune system. It's also a rich source of antioxidants, which help combat inflammation and protect the body from oxidative stress.

Nutritional Information: High in vitamins C, A, and manganese.

14. Cucumber: Cucumber is one of the most hydrating and alkaline vegetables, perfect for detoxifying the body and promoting skin health. Its high-water content helps to flush out toxins and keep the body hydrated, which is key to maintaining alkalinity.

Nutritional Information: Contains vitamin K, silica, and antioxidants.

15. Kale: Kale is a nutrient powerhouse, rich in chlorophyll, antioxidants, and fiber. This leafy green is a staple in the alkaline diet, helping to detoxify the liver, reduce inflammation, and support healthy digestion.

Nutritional Information: Contains vitamins A, C, and K, as well as calcium, potassium, and fiber.

16. Spinach: Spinach is another alkaline green rich in chlorophyll, iron, and antioxidants. It supports bone health, reduces oxidative stress, and helps to maintain healthy blood pressure levels. Its mild flavor makes it a versatile ingredient in juices.

Nutritional Information: High in vitamins A, C, and K, folate, and iron.

17. Celery: Celery is an excellent source of hydration and detoxification, helping to balance the body's pH and reduce acidity. It's rich in vitamins and minerals that support digestion, kidney function, and overall alkalinity.

Nutritional Information: Contains vitamins K, A, and C, potassium, and folate

18. Zucchini: Zucchini is a mild, hydrating vegetable that's great for maintaining an alkaline ph. It's rich in antioxidants and supports digestion and

hydration, making it a perfect base for alkaline juices.

Nutritional Information: Contains vitamin C, potassium, and manganese.

19. Beet Greens: Beet greens are often overlooked but are highly nutritious and alkaline. They're rich in antioxidants, iron, and vitamins that support liver function, detoxification, and cellular repair. They have a slightly bitter taste that blends well with sweeter fruits in juices.

Nutritional Information: High in vitamins A, C, and K, as well as calcium and iron.

20. Dill: Dill is an herb that supports digestion and has anti-inflammatory properties. It's rich in antioxidants and helps reduce oxidative stress, supporting overall health and longevity. Nutritional Information: Contains vitamins A, C, and calcium.

Tips & Best Practices for Juicing

Juicing can be a transformative addition to your health and wellness regimen, particularly when embracing an alkaline lifestyle. However, to truly maximize the benefits of juicing and to ensure a smooth, enjoyable experience, it's essential to adopt some best practices and practical tips. Here are some key insights to help you get the most out of your juicing journey.

1. **Choose Organic Ingredients:** Whenever possible, opt for organic fruits and vegetables. Organic produce is grown without synthetic pesticides and fertilizers, making it a safer and healthier choice for juicing. This commitment not only benefits your health but also supports sustainable agricultural practices.

Dr. Sebi juicing recipes book

2. Incorporate Variety: Variety is the spice of life, and this holds true for your juices as well. Incorporate a wide range of fruits and vegetables to benefit from the diverse nutrients they offer. This not only enhances the flavor of your juices but also ensures that your body receives a broad spectrum of vitamins, minerals, and antioxidants. Think beyond the basics and include less common options like beets, kale, moringa, and cabbage for added nutritional value.

3. Balance Sweetness and Bitterness: When creating juices, aim for a balance between sweet fruits and bitter greens or vegetables. Sweet fruits like apples, oranges, and pineapples can mask the more bitter flavors of greens such as kale, collard greens, or dandelion. This balance not only makes your juices more palatable but also helps maintain a lower glycemic load, keeping your blood sugar levels stable.

4. Prep Your Ingredients: Preparation is key to a seamless juicing experience. Wash your fruits and vegetables thoroughly to remove any dirt, pesticides, or contaminants. For harder vegetables like carrots or beets, chopping them into smaller pieces can make the juicing process easier and more efficient. You might also consider prepping your ingredients ahead of time to make juicing a quick and enjoyable ritual.

5. Stay Hydrated: Juicing is a fantastic way to increase your fluid intake. However, it's important to remember that juices should not replace water. Aim to drink plenty of pure, alkaline water throughout the day in conjunction with your juices. This will help your body stay hydrated and support optimal detoxification.

6. Start Slow: If you're new to juicing or transitioning to an alkaline diet, it's wise to start slowly. Begin with one or two juices a day and gradually increase as your body adapts. This allows your digestive system to adjust and helps prevent potential detox symptoms, such

Dr. Sebi juicing recipes book

as headaches or digestive discomfort.

7. Listen to Your Body: Every individual is unique, and your body may respond differently to certain ingredients. Pay attention to how you feel after consuming different juices. If a particular ingredient doesn't sit well with you, don't hesitate to modify your recipes. Your health journey should be a personal one, tailored to your preferences and needs.

8. Juicing as a Meal Replacement: While juices are packed with nutrients, they can be low in calories. If you're using juices as meal replacements, consider adding ingredients that provide healthy fats or proteins, such as avocado or nut butters, to help make the meal more satiating. This can prevent hunger pangs and provide sustained energy throughout the day.

9. Keep It Fresh: Freshness is key to maximizing the benefits of juicing. Try to consume your juice immediately after preparation to ensure you're getting the most nutrients possible. If you need to store juice for later, keep it in an airtight container and store it in the refrigerator. Even then, aim to consume it within 24 hours to retain the highest nutritional value.

10. Experiment with Herbs and Spices: Don't shy away from incorporating herbs and spices into your juices. Ingredients like ginger, turmeric, cinnamon, and cilantro can enhance the flavor and offer additional health benefits, such as anti-inflammatory properties and digestive support. These little additions can transform a simple juice into a powerful health tonic.

11. Utilize Pulp: Don't discard the pulp leftover from juicing. This byproduct is rich in fiber and nutrients. Consider using it in smoothies, soups, or as a base for vegetable broths.

Incorporating pulp into your meals can help you avoid waste and increase your daily fiber intake.

How to Store and Serve Juices

Storing and serving your freshly made juices properly is essential to preserving their vibrant flavors and nutritional value. When you put in the effort to create nutritious and delicious juices, you want to ensure that they remain as fresh as possible for your enjoyment and health benefits. Here are some detailed guidelines for effectively storing and serving your juices:

1. Use Airtight Containers: When storing juice, the type of container you choose can significantly impact its freshness. opt for glass jars or bottles with tight-fitting lids, as these materials help prevent oxidation, which can degrade the quality of the juice. If possible, use containers made of dark glass to shield your juice from light, which can also contribute to nutrient loss. The goal is to minimize exposure to air and light, both of which can diminish the juice's nutritional profile.

2. Refrigeration is Key: After juicing, always store your juice in the refrigerator to slow down the natural degradation process. Freshly made juice is best consumed immediately, but if you need to store it, aim to keep it in the fridge for no longer than 24 to 48 hours. Although refrigeration extends the shelf life slightly, the nutritional content begins to decline quickly, so it's best to drink it as soon as possible.

3. Fill Containers to the Brim: When transferring juice to your storage container, fill it as much as possible, leaving minimal air space at the top. This technique reduces the amount of air in the container and decreases the chance of oxidation. The less air that is in contact with your juice, the better it will preserve its fresh taste and health benefits.

4. Freeze for Longer Storage: If you want to store your juices for an extended period, consider

freezing them. Freeze juice in ice cube trays, then transfer the frozen cubes into airtight freezer bags for easy access. This method allows you to defrost only what you need while preserving the overall freshness of the remaining juice. Just keep in mind that some separation may occur upon thawing, so give it a good shake or stir before consuming.

5. Serving Your Juices: When it comes time to serve your juice, pour it into a clean glass and enjoy it at your convenience. For a refreshing experience, consider chilling your glassware in the refrigerator prior to serving. You may also garnish your juice with a slice of lemon or a sprig of fresh mint to enhance its presentation and flavor profile. This little touch can elevate the experience, making your juicing ritual feel like a special occasion.

6. Consume with Intent: Juicing is not just about drinking; it's an experience to savor. Take a moment to appreciate the vibrant colors and fresh aromas before taking that first sip. Allow the juice to linger on your palate, paying attention to the intricate flavors and textures. By treating juicing as a mindful practice, you enhance your connection to the nourishment you're providing your body.

Living a Dr. Sebi Lifestyle for Long-Term Health

Transitioning to a Dr. Sebi lifestyle requires commitment, patience, and a willingness to explore the abundance of nature. It invites us to honor our bodies by choosing foods that resonate with our biological makeup, emphasizing the importance of pH balance and the role of nutrients in maintaining cellular health. This lifestyle underscores the value of whole, organic, and non-hybrid foods that provide the body with the essential elements it craves. By adopting this lifestyle, we cultivate a resilient immune system, enhance our vitality, and open ourselves to the healing powers of nature.

Moreover, integrating daily practices such as juicing into our routines allows us to infuse our bodies with concentrated doses of nutrients, supporting our detoxification processes while promoting overall health. Juicing serves as a delicious means to nourish our bodies with essential vitamins, minerals, and antioxidants, which are pivotal for maintaining optimal health. As we savor each sip, we celebrate the vibrant flavors and the life-giving properties of these natural elixirs.

The Dr. Sebi lifestyle encourages us to create a harmonious balance within ourselves, where our physical, emotional, and spiritual aspects align. It invites us to take responsibility for our health, guiding us toward informed food choices that resonate with our values and promote a sustainable way of living. As we cultivate awareness around what we consume, we nurture not only our bodies but also our minds and spirits, leading to a profound transformation in our overall well-being.

Final Thoughts on Juicing and Holistic Health

In this exploration of juicing and holistic health, we have uncovered the incredible potential that lies within the fruits and vegetables that nature generously provides. Juicing is not just a trend; it is a potent practice that empowers us to unlock the healing properties of the foods we consume. By incorporating a variety of nutrient-dense ingredients into our juices, we embark on a path toward improved health, vitality, and longevity.

As we integrate juicing into our daily routines, we become active participants in our health journeys, fostering a relationship with food that is rooted in mindfulness and respect. Each glass of juice serves as a reminder

Dr. Sebi juicing recipes book

of our commitment to nourishing our bodies and honoring the gifts of nature. It is a celebration of the vibrant colors, flavors, and textures that come together to create life-sustaining nourishment.

Ultimately, the journey toward optimal health is unique for each individual, and it is one that is deeply personal. As we embrace the teachings of Dr. Sebi and commit to living a lifestyle that prioritizes alkalinity and whole foods, we step into a world of endless possibilities for wellness. This lifestyle empowers us to transcend the limitations of conventional thinking, to embrace our innate healing abilities, and to cultivate a deeper connection with ourselves and the world around us. As you close this book and step into your own journey, may you be inspired to embrace the power of juicing and holistic health. Remember that your choices matter, and each positive decision contributes to the vibrant tapestry of your life. Celebrate your progress, remain open to learning, and allow the journey of health and wellness to unfold before you in beautiful and transformative ways. Embrace this lifestyle, and witness the remarkable changes it can bring to your life— your body, mind, and spirit will thank you.

Dr. Sebi juicing recipes book

We Value Your Feedback!
Thank you for choosing our book to be part of your journey. Your thoughts and experiences mean the world to us. If this book has inspired, helped, or added value to your life, we would love to hear from you!
Please take a moment to share your review and help others discover the benefits too.

☆ ☆ ☆ ☆ ☆

Simply scan the QR code to leave your feedback.

Made in the USA
Monee, IL
29 March 2025